Neurodegenerative Diseases and the Brain

The Ultimate Guide for Beginners on Causes, Symptoms, and Cutting-Edge Treatments.

(Things You Must Know)

By

Isabella White

Copyright © 2024 by Isabella White.

Disclaimer: *The information in this book is based on the author's research and experiences. It is not intended to replace professional medical advice or treatment. The reader should regularly consult a physician for any health issues and always seek the advice of a physician before modifying diet, supplement, or exercise regimens. The author and publisher shall have neither liability nor responsibility to any person or entity concerning any loss or damage related to the information contained in this book. The information provided is general and may not apply to every individual. Any reliance on the information contained herein is solely at the reader's risk.*

Table of Contents

Introduction..........5

Chapter 1

Understanding Neurodegenerative Diseases............8

What are Neurodegenerative Diseases?..........8

The Complexity of the Brain..........10

The Most Common Neurodegenerative Diseases..........13

Chapter 2

Causes and Risk Factors..........16

Genetic Causes..........16

Environmental Factors..........20

Lifestyle Risks..........23

The Aging Brain..........25

Chapter 3

Early Signs and Symptoms..........29

Memory Loss and Dementia..........29

Motor Impairment..........32

Cognitive Decline..........34

Behavioral and Psychological Symptoms..........35

Chapter 4

Disease Progression and Impact on Brain Function..........38

Stages of Neurodegenerative Diseases..........38

Brain Changes and Degeneration..........41

Chapter 5

Diagnosis and Prognosis..44

Neuropsychological Testing.................................44

Brain Imaging...47

Lumbar Punctures..49

Chapter 6

Treatment Approaches and Their Limitations......... 52

Medications and Therapies..................................52

Side Effects and Risks... 55

Challenges in Treatment..................................... 57

Emerging Treatments.. 59

The Importance of Early Intervention.................62

Chapter 7

Lifestyle Interventions and Supportive Care............ 64

Exercise and Physical Therapy........................... 64

Nutrition and Diet...66

Supportive Care and Services............................. 68

Chapter 8

Supporting Those with Neurodegenerative Diseases... 70

Caregiving Strategies...70

Maintaining Quality of Life.................................73

Legal and Financial Planning..............................75

Communication Tips..77

Conclusion...80

References..83

Resources...84

Introduction

Neurodegenerative diseases are some of the most devastating and perplexing conditions facing both patients and doctors today. These disorders, which include Alzheimer's disease, Parkinson's disease, and Huntington's disease, among others, involve the progressive degeneration and death of neurons in the brain and nervous system.

This neuronal loss leads to declining cognitive, behavioral, and motor function over time. While the causes of most neurodegenerative diseases remain largely unknown, researchers believe a complex interplay between genetic, environmental, and lifestyle factors contributes to their development and progression. Age is the greatest risk factor, with most neurodegenerative disorders occurring in late adulthood.

Receiving a diagnosis of a neurodegenerative disease can be tough and life-altering for patients and their families. In addition to declines in memory, movement, and independence, these disorders also commonly lead to anxiety, depression, and reduced quality of life. Caregivers are also deeply affected as they witness their loved one's gradual loss of function.

Despite major research efforts over the past decades, there are still no cures for these devastating illnesses. Treatment focuses on symptom management via medications and therapies aimed at improving daily function and quality of life. However, the efficacy of available interventions remains limited.

It is clear we still have far to go in our understanding of neurodegenerative disease pathology and how to treat these conditions effectively. This book aims to provide readers with a comprehensive overview of our current knowledge regarding common neurodegenerative disorders.

In the following chapters, we will explore the suspected causes and risk factors for conditions like Alzheimer's and Parkinson's diseases. We will also dive into the clinical presentation, diagnosis, disease course, and management strategies. Cutting-edge research on novel treatments and preventative approaches will also be discussed.

This book will empower readers with the information they need to understand these complex diseases better. My goal is to present the latest scientific findings in an accessible way for patients, caregivers, and healthcare professionals seeking to stay up-to-date on neurodegenerative disease treatment and research. While many mysteries remain, arming ourselves with knowledge puts us in the best position to cope with and overcome these challenging illnesses.

Chapter 1

Understanding Neurodegenerative Diseases

What are Neurodegenerative Diseases?

Neurodegenerative diseases are a group of disorders that affect the structure and function of the brain and nervous system. They are characterized by the progressive loss of neurons, the cells that transmit and process information in the brain and other parts of the nervous system.

As neurons die or become damaged, they cause various symptoms, such as cognitive impairment, memory loss, movement disorders, mood changes, and sensory problems.

Some of the most common neurodegenerative diseases are Alzheimer's disease, Parkinson's disease, Huntington's disease, amyotrophic lateral sclerosis (ALS), and multiple sclerosis (MS). These diseases have different causes, risk factors, and manifestations, but they share some common features and challenges.

For example, they are all incurable, chronic, and debilitating; they affect millions of people worldwide and impose a huge burden on individuals, families, and society; and they have no definitive diagnosis, prevention, or treatment. The exact mechanisms of neurodegeneration are not fully understood. Still, researchers have identified some possible factors that contribute to the onset and progression of these diseases.

These include genetic mutations, environmental toxins, oxidative stress, inflammation, protein aggregation, mitochondrial dysfunction, and impaired cellular communication. Understanding these factors and how they interact with each other is crucial for developing new strategies to cope with and overcome neurodegenerative diseases.

The Complexity of the Brain

The brain is the most complex and fascinating organ in the human body. It is composed of billions of neurons and trillions of connections that enable us to think, feel, learn, remember, and perform countless other functions. The brain is also the control center of the nervous system, which regulates all the body's activities, such as breathing, heartbeat, digestion, movement, and sensation.

The brain comprises three main parts: the cerebrum, the cerebellum, and the brainstem. The cerebrum, being the largest part of the brain, is divided into two hemispheres connected by the corpus callosum. It is responsible for higher cognitive functions such as language, reasoning, problem-solving, creativity, and emotion.

The cerebrum is also divided into four lobes: the frontal lobe, the parietal lobe, the temporal lobe, and the occipital lobe. Each lobe has specific functions and processes different types of information.

The cerebellum is located at the back of the brain and coordinates movement, balance, posture, and coordination. The cerebellum also plays a role in learning, memory, and cognition. The brainstem is the lowest part of the brain and connects the brain to the spinal cord.

The brainstem controls vital functions such as breathing, heartbeat, blood pressure, and sleep. The brainstem also contains several structures that are involved in sensory and motor pathways, such as the thalamus, the hypothalamus, the midbrain, the pons, and the medulla oblongata.

The brain is also composed of different types of cells, such as neurons, glia, and blood vessels. Neurons are the basic units of the nervous system, and they communicate with each other through electrical and chemical signals. Neurons have three main parts: the cell body, the axon, and the dendrites. The cell body contains the nucleus and other organelles that support the neuron's function.

The axon is a long projection that carries signals away from the cell body to other neurons or target cells. The dendrites are short branches that receive signals from other neurons or sensory stimuli. Neurons form complex networks and circuits that underlie the brain's functions and behaviors.

Glia are the supporting cells of the nervous system and outnumber neurons by about 10 to 1. Glia has various roles, such as providing structural and metabolic support, maintaining the blood-brain barrier, modulating synaptic transmission, and participating in immune and inflammatory responses. Some of the main types of glia are astrocytes, oligodendrocytes, microglia, and ependymal cells.

Blood vessels are the tubes that transport blood throughout the body and the brain. The blood carries oxygen, nutrients, hormones, and waste products to and from the brain. The brain consumes about 20%

of the body's oxygen and glucose despite accounting for only 2% of the body's weight.

The cerebral circulation is a network of cerebral arteries, veins, and capillaries that regulates the blood supply to the brain. The cerebral circulation is also connected to the systemic circulation, which distributes blood to the rest of the body.

The brain is a remarkable organ that enables us to experience and interact with the world. However, the brain is also vulnerable to various diseases and disorders that can impair its function and structure.

The Most Common Neurodegenerative Diseases

The most prevalent neurodegenerative diseases are Alzheimer's disease, Parkinson's disease, and amyotrophic lateral sclerosis (ALS). These conditions stand out for both their prevalence and the extensive neuronal degeneration they cause.

Alzheimer's disease is arguably the most infamous neurodegenerative disorder. It accounts for up to

70% of dementia cases. Pathologically, Alzheimer's involves the accumulation of toxic protein clusters called beta-amyloid plaques and tau tangles within neurons. This provokes widespread cortical atrophy and the steady destruction of memory, cognition, and personality.

Parkinson's disease, on the other hand, selectively targets dopamine-producing neurons in the midbrain. The hallmark symptoms of Parkinson's are motor impairments like tremors, rigidity, and slowed movements. These result from the loss of dopaminergic neurons in brain areas regulating motor control. Parkinson's also features abnormal clumping of the alpha-synuclein protein inside neurons.

Amyotrophic lateral sclerosis, or ALS, affects both upper and lower motor neurons, destroying the nerve cells that control voluntary muscle movements. ALS causes muscle weakness, paralysis, and ultimately respiratory failure due to denervation. It is rapidly fatal, with most patients surviving just 2 to 5 years after diagnosis.

While Alzheimer's, Parkinson's, and ALS have distinct clinical courses and neuropathologies, they share disease mechanisms like inflammation and protein aggregation that lead to neurodegeneration. However, factors like aging and genetics also influence individual risk. For instance, ALS peaks earlier than Alzheimer's or Parkinson's, frequently striking patients in mid-adulthood.

These major neurodegenerative diseases have a devastating impact on quality of life and independence. Currently, available treatments only marginally slow their progression. Finding ways to halt neurodegeneration remains one of the foremost challenges in medicine and neuroscience. Successful therapies may need to target mechanisms common across multiple neurodegenerative conditions for maximal benefit.

Chapter 2

Causes and Risk Factors

Genetic Causes

Genetic causes are one factor that can contribute to the development of neurodegenerative diseases. Some neurodegenerative diseases are inherited in a Mendelian fashion, meaning that they are caused by mutations in a single gene that are passed down from one or both parents.

These diseases are usually rare and have an early onset. Examples of these diseases are Huntington's disease, familial Alzheimer's disease, familial Parkinson's disease, and some forms of spinocerebellar ataxia.

Other neurodegenerative diseases are influenced by multiple genes that interact with each other and with environmental factors. These diseases are more common and have a later onset. Examples of these diseases are sporadic Alzheimer's disease, sporadic Parkinson's disease, and amyotrophic lateral sclerosis. These diseases are not directly inherited, but they have a genetic component that affects the risk and severity of the disease.

Genetic studies have identified many genes that are associated with neurodegenerative diseases. These genes encode proteins that are involved in various cellular processes, such as protein folding, degradation, trafficking, and aggregation; mitochondrial function and energy metabolism; oxidative stress and inflammation; synaptic function and neurotransmission; and cell survival and death.

Mutations or variations in these genes can disrupt the normal function of these proteins and cause neuronal damage or death. Some of the genes that have been linked to neurodegenerative diseases are listed below:

- **APP, PSEN1, and PSEN2:** These genes are involved in the production of amyloid-beta, a protein that forms plaques in the brains of Alzheimer's disease patients. Mutations in these genes cause familial Alzheimer's disease, a rare and early-onset form of the disease.

- **APOE:** This gene encodes apolipoprotein E, a protein that transports cholesterol and lipids in the blood and brain. The APOE gene has three common variants: APOE2, APOE3, and APOE4. The APOE4 variant is associated with an increased risk of sporadic Alzheimer's disease, the most common and late-onset form of the disease.

- **SNCA:** This gene encodes alpha-synuclein, a protein that is abundant in the brain and plays a role in synaptic function. Mutations or duplications of this gene cause familial Parkinson's disease, a rare and early-onset form of the disease. Alpha-synuclein also forms aggregates called Lewy bodies in the brains of Parkinson's disease patients.

- **LRRK2:** This gene creates the protein leucine-rich repeat kinase 2, which helps cells do many things, like moving the cytoskeleton, moving vesicles, and cleaning up dead cells. Mutations in this gene are the most common cause of familial Parkinson's disease and also increase the risk of sporadic Parkinson's disease.

- **SOD1, TARDBP, and C9orf72:** These genes encode superoxide dismutase 1, TAR DNA-binding protein 43, and chromosome 9 open reading frame 72, respectively. These proteins are involved in various cellular functions, such as oxidative stress, RNA metabolism, and autophagy. Mutations in these genes are the most common causes of familial amyotrophic lateral sclerosis. This rare and fatal neurodegenerative disease affects the motor neurons.

Environmental Factors

Environmental factors are another factor that can contribute to the development of neurodegenerative diseases. Some environmental factors are natural, such as air pollution, water contamination, and soil quality. Others are artificial, such as pesticides, metals, solvents, and electromagnetic fields.

Exposure to these factors can affect the brain and the nervous system in various ways, such as by causing oxidative stress, inflammation, mitochondrial dysfunction, and epigenetic changes. Environmental factors can also interact with genetic factors and modulate the risk and severity of neurodegenerative diseases.

Some of the environmental factors that have been associated with neurodegenerative diseases are listed below:

- **Pesticides, fungicides, and insecticides:** These are chemicals used to control pests and weeds in agriculture and other settings. Exposure to these chemicals can damage the nervous system and increase the risk of Parkinson's disease, Alzheimer's disease, and amyotrophic lateral sclerosis.

- **Metals:** These are elements that are found in the earth's crust and can be released into the environment by natural or human activities. Some metals, such as iron, copper, and zinc, are essential for the normal function of the brain and the nervous system. However, excessive or deficient levels of these metals can cause neurotoxicity and neurodegeneration. Other metals, such as lead, mercury, arsenic, and manganese, are toxic to the nervous system and can cause cognitive impairment, movement disorders, and neurodegeneration.

- **Solvents:** These are substances that are used to dissolve or extract other substances, such as paints, adhesives, degreasers, and cleaners. Exposure to these substances can affect the nervous system and cause headaches, dizziness, memory loss, and neurodegeneration. Some solvents, such as toluene, benzene, and trichloroethylene, have been linked to Parkinson's disease, Alzheimer's disease, and multiple system atrophy.

- **Electromagnetic fields:** These are invisible fields of energy that are produced by electric currents and magnetic materials. Exposure to these fields can occur from natural sources, such as the earth's magnetic field, or artificial sources, such as power lines, appliances, and wireless devices. The effects of electromagnetic fields on the nervous system are controversial and not well understood. Some studies have suggested that exposure to electromagnetic fields may increase the risk of Alzheimer's disease, amyotrophic lateral sclerosis, and multiple system atrophy. However, other studies have found no association or even protective effects.

Lifestyle Risks

Lifestyle risks are another factor that can contribute to the development of neurodegenerative diseases. Lifestyle risks are habits or behaviors that can affect the health and well-being of the brain and the nervous system. Some lifestyle risks include:

- **Physical inactivity:** Physical activity is beneficial for the brain and the nervous system, as it improves blood flow, oxygen delivery, glucose metabolism, and neuroplasticity. Physical activity also reduces the risk of cardiovascular and cerebrovascular diseases, which can damage the brain and cause neurodegeneration. Studies have shown that physical inactivity is associated with an increased risk of Alzheimer's disease, Parkinson's disease, and amyotrophic lateral sclerosis.

- **Unhealthy diet:** Diet is important for the brain and the nervous system, as it provides essential nutrients, antioxidants, and anti-inflammatory compounds. The diet also influences the gut microbiota, which can affect the brain and the nervous system through the gut-brain axis. Studies have shown that unhealthy diets, such as high-fat, high-sugar, or low-fiber diets, are associated with an increased risk of Alzheimer's disease, Parkinson's disease, and multiple sclerosis.

- **Alcohol and tobacco use:** Alcohol and tobacco are harmful substances that can damage the brain and the nervous system, as they cause oxidative stress, inflammation, mitochondrial dysfunction, and epigenetic changes. Alcohol and tobacco also interfere with the normal function of neurotransmitters, hormones, and enzymes. Studies have shown that alcohol and tobacco use are associated with an increased risk of Alzheimer's disease, Parkinson's disease, and multiple system atrophy.

The Aging Brain

The term aging brain refers to the changes that occur in the brain as people age. These changes can affect the brain's structure, function, and cognition. Some of the changes are normal and inevitable, while others are abnormal and associated with diseases.

Some of the normal changes that happen to the aging brain are:

- **Brain shrinkage:** The brain tends to lose volume and weight as people age, especially in the frontal lobe, the temporal lobe, and the hippocampus. These regions are involved in executive functions, memory, and learning.

- **White matter changes:** The white matter is the part of the brain that contains myelinated axons, which connect different brain regions and transmit signals. The myelin sheath, which insulates and protects the axons, can degrade or deteriorate with age, causing slower processing speed and reduced cognitive performance.

- **Reduced blood flow:** The blood vessels that supply the brain with oxygen and nutrients can narrow or become less flexible with age, reducing the blood flow to the brain. This can impair the brain's function and increase the risk of stroke.

- **Neurotransmitter changes:** The neurotransmitters are the chemicals that enable communication between neurons. The levels and activity of some neurotransmitters, such as dopamine, serotonin, and acetylcholine, can decline with age, affecting mood, motivation, attention, and memory.

Some of the abnormal changes that can happen to the aging brain are:

- **Neurodegeneration:** This is the progressive loss of neurons and synapses, which can lead to cognitive impairment, dementia, and neurodegenerative diseases such as Alzheimer's, Parkinson's, and amyotrophic lateral sclerosis. The causes and mechanisms of neurodegeneration are not fully understood, but they may involve genetic, environmental, and lifestyle factors.

- **Neuroinflammation:** This is the activation of the immune system in the brain, which infections, injuries, or diseases can trigger. Neuroinflammation can have beneficial or detrimental effects on the brain, depending on the type, duration, and intensity of the response. Chronic or excessive neuroinflammation can damage the brain and contribute to neurodegeneration and cognitive decline.

- **Protein aggregation:** This is the accumulation of abnormal or misfolded proteins in the brain, which can interfere with the normal function of neurons and synapses. Different neurodegenerative diseases are characterized by different types of protein aggregates, such as amyloid-beta plaques and tau tangles in Alzheimer's disease, alpha-synuclein Lewy bodies in Parkinson's disease, and TDP-43 inclusions in amyotrophic lateral sclerosis.

The aging brain is a complex and dynamic organ that undergoes various changes throughout the lifespan. Some of these changes are inevitable and may not affect the quality of life. In contrast, others are preventable or treatable and may impair the cognitive abilities and well-being of older adults.

Chapter 3

Early Signs and Symptoms

Memory Loss and Dementia

Memory loss and dementia are two related but distinct concepts that can affect older adults. Memory loss is the inability to remember information, events, or experiences that were previously stored in the brain.

Dementia is a general term for a decline in cognitive abilities, such as memory, thinking, reasoning, and language that interferes with daily functioning. Memory loss is one of the most common symptoms of dementia, but not all memory loss is caused by dementia. There are different types and causes of memory loss and dementia. Some of the most common ones are:

- **Age-related memory loss:** This is a normal part of aging that affects everyone to some degree. It involves minor and occasional forgetfulness, such as misplacing keys or forgetting names or appointments. It does not affect the ability to learn new things, communicate, or perform daily tasks.

- **Mild cognitive impairment (MCI):** This is a condition that involves more noticeable and frequent memory problems than normal aging but is not severe enough to be diagnosed as dementia. It affects about 15–25% of people over 65 years old. People with MCI may have trouble remembering recent events, following conversations, or finding words. They may also have difficulties with other cognitive functions, such as planning, organizing, or decision-making. MCI does not significantly impair daily functioning, but it increases the risk of developing dementia in the future.

- **Alzheimer's disease:** This is the most common cause of dementia, accounting for 60–80% of all cases. It is a progressive and irreversible brain disease that destroys neurons and synapses, leading to cognitive decline and behavioral changes. It affects about 6 million people in the United States and 50 million people worldwide. People with Alzheimer's disease have problems with memory, language, judgment, orientation, and reasoning. They may also experience mood swings, agitation, confusion, hallucinations, and delusions. Alzheimer's disease worsens over time and eventually affects all aspects of daily living.

- **Vascular dementia:** This is the second most common cause of dementia, accounting for 10–20% of all cases. It is caused by reduced blood flow to the brain due to strokes, mini-strokes, or other vascular problems. It affects about 3 million people in the United States and 10 million people worldwide. People with vascular dementia have problems with memory, attention, executive functions, and visuospatial skills. They may also have physical symptoms, such as weakness, numbness, or difficulty walking. Vascular dementia can occur suddenly or gradually, depending on the type and extent of the brain damage.

Other conditions can affect memory and cognition, such as Parkinson's disease, Lewy body dementia, frontotemporal dementia, traumatic brain injury, infections, tumors, medications, and depression.

Motor Impairment

Motor impairment is a term that refers to the partial or total loss of function of a body part, usually a limb or limbs. This may result in muscle weakness, poor stamina, a lack of muscle control, or total paralysis. Motor impairment can be caused by various factors, such as trauma, disease, or congenital conditions, that affect the brain, the spinal cord, or the peripheral nerves. Some examples of motor impairment are:

- **Cerebral palsy:** This is a group of disorders that affect the movement and posture of a person due to damage or abnormal development of the brain before, during, or after birth. People with cerebral palsy may have difficulty with balance, coordination, speech, and learning. The severity and type of cerebral palsy can vary widely among individuals.

- **Parkinson's disease:** This is a progressive and degenerative disorder that affects the nerve cells in the brain that produce dopamine, a chemical that regulates movement and emotion. People with Parkinson's disease may experience tremors, rigidity, slowness of movement, and difficulty with walking and balance. They may also have cognitive and emotional problems, such as depression, anxiety, and dementia.

- **Stroke:** This is a sudden interruption of blood flow to the brain due to a clot or a burst vessel that deprives the brain cells of oxygen and nutrients. This can cause damage or death to the affected brain cells, leading to impaired function and communication. People who suffer a stroke may have weakness or paralysis on one side of the body, difficulty with speech, vision, and memory, and changes in mood and behavior.

Cognitive Decline

Cognitive decline refers to the deterioration of mental abilities such as memory, attention, reasoning, and language. It can be a normal part of aging or a sign of a more severe condition, such as dementia or Alzheimer's disease.

Cognitive decline can affect the quality of life and well-being of the affected person and their caregivers. Some of the signs and symptoms of cognitive decline are:

- Difficulty remembering recent events, names, or appointments

- Trouble following instructions, directions, or conversations
- Losing track of time, date, or place
- Making poor decisions or judgments
- Having trouble finding words or expressing thoughts
- Experiencing mood swings, anxiety, or depression
- Losing interest in or motivation in once enjoyable activities

Behavioral and Psychological Symptoms

Behavioral and psychological symptoms are common in people with neurodegenerative diseases, especially in their advanced stages. These symptoms can affect the mood, personality, behavior, and cognition of the affected person and cause distress and challenges for the person and their caregivers.

Some of the behavioral and psychological symptoms that can occur in neurodegenerative diseases are:

- **Depression:** This is a persistent feeling of sadness, hopelessness, or emptiness that interferes with daily functioning and enjoyment of life. Depression can affect up to 50% of people with Alzheimer's disease, Parkinson's disease, and amyotrophic lateral sclerosis.

- **Anxiety:** This is a feeling of nervousness, worry, or fear that is excessive or disproportionate to the situation. Anxiety can affect up to 40% of people with Alzheimer's disease, Parkinson's disease, and multiple sclerosis.

- **Apathy:** This is a lack of interest, motivation, or emotion for activities or people that were once enjoyable or meaningful. Apathy can affect up to 70% of people with Alzheimer's disease, Parkinson's disease, and frontotemporal dementia.

- **Agitation:** This is a state of restlessness, irritability, or aggression that internal or external factors, such as pain, boredom, frustration, or environmental changes, can trigger. Agitation can affect up to 80% of people with Alzheimer's disease, Parkinson's disease, and Huntington's disease.

- **Psychosis:** This is a loss of contact with reality that can involve hallucinations (seeing, hearing, or feeling things that are not there) or delusions (false beliefs that are not based on evidence). Psychosis can affect up to 50% of people with Alzheimer's disease, Parkinson's disease, and Lewy body dementia.

Chapter 4

Disease Progression and Impact on Brain Function

Stages of Neurodegenerative Diseases

Neurodegenerative diseases are a group of disorders that affect the brain and the nervous system, causing progressive loss of neurons and synapses. These diseases have different causes, symptoms, and treatments, but they also share some common features and challenges.

One of these features is that they tend to progress in stages, from mild to severe, over time. The stages of neurodegenerative diseases can vary depending on the type and severity of the disease. Still, they generally follow a similar pattern:

- **Preclinical stage:** This is the earliest stage of the disease when there are no noticeable symptoms, but there are already some changes in the brain that biomarkers or imaging tests can detect. This stage can last for years or even decades before the onset of clinical symptoms.

- **Mild stage:** This is the stage when the first signs and symptoms of the disease appear, such as memory loss, cognitive impairment, movement problems, or behavioral changes. These symptoms are usually mild and do not interfere significantly with daily functioning. Still, they may affect the quality of life and well-being of the affected person and their caregivers. This stage can last for months or years, depending on the disease and the treatment.

- **Moderate stage:** This is the stage when the symptoms of the disease become more noticeable and severe, affecting multiple domains of cognition, behavior, and function. The affected person may have difficulty with language, reasoning, judgment, orientation, and visuospatial skills. They may also experience mood swings, agitation, psychosis, or sleep problems. They may need assistance with some activities of daily living, such as dressing, bathing, or eating. This stage can last for months or years, depending on the disease and the treatment.

- **Severe stage:** This is the final stage of the disease, when the symptoms of the disease are very severe and debilitating, affecting all aspects of daily living. The affected person may lose the ability to communicate, recognize people or objects, or control their bodily functions. They may also suffer from infections, malnutrition, or other complications. They may need constant care and supervision, either at home or in a facility. This stage can last for months or years until death.

The stages of neurodegenerative diseases are not fixed or rigid but rather fluid and dynamic. They can overlap, fluctuate, or vary among individuals and populations. Therefore, it is important to monitor the progression of the disease and adjust care and support accordingly.

Brain Changes and Degeneration

Brain changes and degeneration are terms that describe the alterations in the structure and function of the brain that occur due to various factors, such as aging, disease, injury, or environment. These changes can affect the size, shape, connectivity, and activity of the brain cells and regions, leading to cognitive, behavioral, and physical impairments.

Some of the common causes of brain changes and degeneration are:

- **Aging:** As people age, the brain undergoes normal changes, such as brain shrinkage, white matter changes, reduced blood flow, and neurotransmitter changes. These changes can affect memory, attention, processing speed, and executive functions. Still, they do not necessarily impair daily functioning or quality of life. However, some people may experience more severe and abnormal changes than expected for their age, which can lead to cognitive decline or dementia.

- **Neurodegenerative diseases:** These are a group of disorders that cause progressive and irreversible loss of neurons and synapses, resulting in cognitive decline and dementia. Some of the most common neurodegenerative diseases are Alzheimer's disease, Parkinson's disease, Huntington's disease, and amyotrophic lateral sclerosis. These diseases have different causes, symptoms, and treatments. Still, they share some common mechanisms, such as neuroinflammation, protein aggregation, and oxidative stress.

- **Traumatic brain injury:** This is sudden damage to the brain caused by an external force, such as a fall, a car accident, or a gunshot wound. Traumatic brain injury can cause bleeding, swelling, or bruising of the brain, leading to impaired function and communication. Depending on the location and severity of the injury, a traumatic brain injury can cause memory loss, cognitive impairment, mood changes, or motor problems.

- **Environmental factors:** Exposure to toxins, pollutants, or infections can affect the brain and the nervous system, causing oxidative stress, inflammation, mitochondrial dysfunction, and epigenetic changes. These factors can interact with genetic and lifestyle factors and modulate the risk and severity of brain changes and degeneration. Some of the environmental factors that have been associated with brain changes and degeneration are pesticides, metals, solvents, and electromagnetic fields.

Chapter 5

Diagnosis and Prognosis

Neuropsychological Testing

Neuropsychological testing is a critical component of diagnosing and assessing neurodegenerative diseases. These standardized tests evaluate cognitive domains commonly impacted by neurodegeneration, like memory, executive function, language, and visuospatial skills.

Testing helps determine a patient's cognitive profile and deficits, clarifying which brain networks are affected. For example, poor performance on memory tasks indicates hippocampal damage, while executive dysfunction points to frontal lobe pathology.

Tests also detect subtle cognitive changes early in disease progression, often before symptoms are overt. Detecting early neuropsychological deficits affords opportunities for timely interventions to preserve function. For progressive conditions like Alzheimer's disease, repeated testing over time tracks disease advancement.

There are two main categories of neuropsychological tests. General screening evaluations include commonly used batteries like the Mini-Mental State Exam (MMSE), which tests multiple domains. Poor scores prompt more detailed testing.

Domain-specific batteries deeply probe particular cognitive functions. For instance, memory tests like word-list learning assess declarative memory mediated by the hippocampus. Executive function tests require skills like organization, multitasking, and impulse control.

Ideal diagnostic batteries cover several cognitive domains. Testing both general cognition and specific areas provides the clearest snapshot of a patient's strengths, weaknesses, and frontal versus posterior brain function.

Skilled neuropsychologists interpret results in a holistic, patient-centered manner. They consider factors like age, education, and cultural background that influence "normal" cognitive performance. Results are integrated with clinical history, neuroimaging, and lab findings to derive insights into disease processes affecting the brain.

Like all tests, neuropsychological evaluations have limitations. Performance can be impacted by physical disabilities, anxiety, medications, and poor effort unrelated to neuropathology. Also, available tests may not keep pace with rapidly evolving research on brain function networks.

Overall, neuropsychological testing remains the gold standard for objectively and precisely capturing the real-world cognitive impacts of neurodegeneration.

Quantifying cognitive status aids diagnosis, gauges progression, and determines the best strategies for maximizing patient function and independence.

Brain Imaging

Neuroimaging techniques like MRI and PET scans visually reveal the damaging effects of neurodegeneration on brain structure and function. Imaging can detect changes early, even before symptoms appear. Different modalities provide complementary information to pinpoint disease locations and monitor advancement.

Structural MRI scans delineate gross cerebral atrophy reflective of neuronal loss. This technique excels at capturing widespread cortical degeneration in Alzheimer's disease. MRIs detect hippocampal and temporal lobe shrinkage associated with early Alzheimer's-related memory loss.

Functional MRI (fMRI) maps neural activity by measuring blood flow. It shows how brain activation patterns change with neurodegeneration. fMRIs also aid in presurgical planning to avoid damaging the eloquent cortex.

PET imaging uses radioactive tracers to quantify metabolism, blood flow, and protein deposition. It visualizes early hypometabolism indicative of Alzheimer's and Parkinson's diseases. PET also reveals Alzheimer's-related amyloid plaques and tau tangles years before symptom onset.

Molecular PET tracers like Pittsburgh Compound B (PiB) selectively bind beta-amyloid. High PiB retention predicts later dementia development. Tau PET tracers also recently emerged to image Alzheimer's tau burden.

PET imaging of dopamine transporters mirrors dopamine nerve terminal loss in Parkinson's disease. This aids in differentiating Parkinsonian syndromes.

Hybrid PET/MRI scanners fuse PET molecular imaging with MRI's structural detail. Compared to PET/CT, PET/MRI improves scan accuracy and reduces radiation exposure.

Nevertheless, no individual imaging modality provides a complete picture. Multimodal imaging, combining techniques like MRI, PET, and CT, best captures all facets of neurodegeneration. Fusing images also enhances diagnostic and prognostic accuracy.

Overall, neuroimaging elucidates neurodegenerative disease progression in living patients. Images deliver objective visual evidence to confirm clinical impressions. Longitudinal imaging over the years may one day aid in personalized prognosis and treatment monitoring if interventions become available to slow these conditions.

Lumbar Punctures

A lumbar puncture, also known as a spinal tap, is a procedure that obtains cerebrospinal fluid (CSF) for analysis. In neurodegenerative disease diagnosis, lumbar punctures provide insight into brain biochemistry and protein markers indicative of specific conditions.

During a lumbar puncture, a hollow needle is inserted between vertebrae in the lower spine to access the CSF-filled subarachnoid space. Approximately 10–20 mL of CSF is collected for laboratory testing. This fluid bathes the brain and spinal cord, making it an excellent proxy for central nervous system biochemistry.

Several Alzheimer's disease biomarkers are reliably measured in the CSF. Low levels of amyloid beta reflect accumulation in plaques. Elevated tau and phosphorylated tau indicate tangle pathology. The amyloid/tau ratio predicts Alzheimer's onset and progression.

In Parkinson's disease, reduced CSF dopamine metabolite levels parallel nigrostriatal neuron loss. Alpha-synuclein, the protein that misfolds in Parkinson's, is also detectable.

CSF analysis aids differential diagnosis. For example, normal tau distinguishes Alzheimer's from frontotemporal dementia, and specific CSF inflammatory profiles distinguish neurodegenerative diseases from autoimmune disorders like multiple sclerosis.

Lumbar punctures are relatively safe outpatient procedures. However, potential side effects include headaches, infections, and bleeding. Factors like diurnal variation in biomarker levels also limit CSF testing.

Looking ahead, improved CSF biomarkers could enable earlier diagnosis and tracking of neurodegenerative disease. Optimizing lumbar puncture protocols and data interpretation may expand the utility of CSF analysis.

Ultimately, lumbar punctures provide a sample of the brain's internal milieu in living patients. CSF testing delivers insights unobtainable through imaging or cognitive testing alone. When paired with clinical evaluation and neuropsychological profiling, it becomes a powerful diagnostic tool for unraveling complex neurodegenerative diseases.

Chapter 6

Treatment Approaches and Their Limitations

Medications and Therapies

Neurodegenerative diseases are currently incurable and have limited treatment options. Most of the medications and therapies that are available aim to relieve the symptoms, slow down the progression, or improve the quality of life of the affected person and their caregivers. However, these treatments have various limitations, such as side effects, low efficacy, high cost, or accessibility issues.

Some of the medications and therapies that are used for neurodegenerative diseases are:

- **Cholinesterase inhibitors:** These drugs inhibit the enzyme that breaks down acetylcholine, a neurotransmitter involved in memory and learning. They are used to treat mild to moderate Alzheimer's disease and some forms of dementia. They can help improve cognitive function and delay the decline of memory and thinking. However, they have side effects, such as nausea, vomiting, diarrhea, and weight loss. They also do not stop the underlying disease process or prevent the eventual loss of neurons and synapses.

- **Dopamine agonists:** These are drugs that mimic the action of dopamine, a neurotransmitter involved in movement and emotion. They are used to treat Parkinson's disease and some forms of dementia. They can help reduce the symptoms of tremor, rigidity, and slowness of movement. However, they have side effects such as nausea, drowsiness, hallucinations, and compulsive behaviors. They also do not stop the underlying disease process or prevent the eventual loss of neurons and synapses.

- **Riluzole:** This is a drug that modulates the activity of glutamate, a neurotransmitter involved in excitatory signaling. It is used to treat amyotrophic lateral sclerosis, a fatal neurodegenerative disease that affects motor neurons. It can help prolong survival by a few months and delay the need for mechanical ventilation. However, it has side effects such as nausea, dizziness, liver toxicity, and blood disorders. It also does not stop the underlying disease process or prevent the eventual loss of neurons and synapses.

- **Stem cell therapy:** This is a therapy that involves the transplantation of stem cells, which are cells that can differentiate into various types of cells, into the brain or the spinal cord. It is used to treat various neurodegenerative diseases, such as Alzheimer's disease, Parkinson's disease, Huntington's disease, and spinal cord injury. It can help to replace lost or damaged neurons and synapses, restore the function and communication of the nervous system, and enhance the regeneration and repair of the brain tissue. However, it has limitations, such as ethical issues, safety concerns, technical challenges, and regulatory barriers. It also requires further research and development to prove its efficacy and feasibility.

Side Effects and Risks

Side effects and risks are the potential negative consequences of using medications and therapies for neurodegenerative diseases. These can vary depending on the type, dose, duration, and combination of the treatment, as well as the individual characteristics and conditions of the patient. Some of the common side effects and risks are:

- **Nausea, vomiting, diarrhea, and weight loss:** These are gastrointestinal symptoms that can occur with cholinesterase inhibitors, dopamine agonists, and riluzole. They can affect the patient's appetite, hydration, and nutrition.

- **Drowsiness, dizziness, and falls:** These are neurological symptoms that can occur with cholinesterase inhibitors, dopamine agonists, and riluzole. They can affect the alertness, balance, and coordination of the patient.

- **Hallucinations, delusions, and compulsive behaviors:** These are psychiatric symptoms that can occur with dopamine agonists. They can affect the perception, cognition, and emotions of the patient.

- **Liver toxicity and blood disorders:** These are systemic symptoms that can occur with riluzole. They can affect the function and health of the liver and blood cells.

- **Ethical issues:** These are moral and social concerns that can arise with stem cell therapy. They can involve the source, manipulation, and use of stem cells, as well as the rights, consent, and safety of the donors and recipients.

- **Safety concerns:** These are medical and technical challenges that can arise with stem cell therapy. They can involve the quality, purity, and compatibility of the stem cells, as well as the risk of infection, rejection, or tumor formation.

Challenges in Treatment

Treatment for neurodegenerative diseases is a challenging and complex task, as many factors affect the development, progression, and outcome of these diseases. Some of the challenges in treatment are:

- Lack of understanding of the causes and mechanisms of neurodegeneration: Despite the advances in neuroscience research, the exact causes and mechanisms of neurodegeneration still need to be fully understood. This limits the ability to identify and target the key molecular and cellular events that trigger or drive the disease process.

- Lack of reliable biomarkers and diagnostic tools: Biomarkers are measurable indicators of the presence, severity, or progression of a disease. Diagnostic tools are methods or devices that can detect or measure biomarkers. Biomarkers and diagnostic tools are essential for the early and accurate diagnosis, prognosis, and monitoring of neurodegenerative diseases. However, few biomarkers and diagnostic tools are validated, specific, and sensitive to neurodegenerative diseases.

- Lack of effective and safe treatments: Most of the current treatments for neurodegenerative diseases are symptomatic, meaning that they only relieve the symptoms but do not stop or reverse the underlying disease process. Moreover, these treatments have various limitations, such as side effects, low efficacy, high cost, or accessibility issues. Few treatments are disease-modifying, meaning that they can slow down, halt, or reverse neurodegeneration.

- Lack of patient and caregiver involvement and support: Patients and caregivers are the most important stakeholders in the treatment of neurodegenerative diseases, as they are directly affected by the disease and its impact on their quality of life and well-being. However, they often face challenges such as stigma, isolation, discrimination, or a lack of information, education, or resources. They also have diverse and unmet needs, preferences, and expectations, which the current healthcare system may not adequately address.

Emerging Treatments

Emerging treatments are new and innovative approaches that aim to treat or cure neurodegenerative diseases by targeting the underlying causes and mechanisms of neurodegeneration. Some of the emerging treatments that are being developed and tested for neurodegenerative diseases are:

- **Immunotherapy:** This is a treatment that involves the use of the immune system or its components to fight the disease. Immunotherapy can take various forms, such as vaccines, antibodies, or cell-based therapies. Immunotherapy can help to clear the toxic proteins that accumulate in the brain, such as amyloid beta or alpha-synuclein, or modulate the inflammatory response that contributes to neurodegeneration.

- **Gene therapy:** This is a treatment that involves the delivery of genetic material to the cells or tissues to correct or modify the expression of a gene involved in the disease. Gene therapy can use various vectors, such as viruses, nanoparticles, or liposomes, to transfer the genetic material. Gene therapy can help restore the function of a defective or missing gene or silence or edit a harmful gene that affects the survival or function of neurons or synapses.

- **Neuroprotection:** This is a treatment that involves the use of drugs or molecules that can protect the neurons and synapses from damage or death. Neuroprotection can target various pathways, such as oxidative stress, mitochondrial dysfunction, or apoptosis, that are involved in neurodegeneration. Neuroprotection can help to prevent or delay the loss of neurons or synapses and preserve the function and structure of the brain and the nervous system.

These are the emerging treatments that are being developed and tested for neurodegenerative diseases. Many more treatments are based on different approaches, such as neurorestoration, neurorehabilitation, or nanotechnology, that aim to treat or cure neurodegenerative diseases.

These treatments are promising and exciting, but they also face various challenges, such as ethical issues, safety concerns, technical difficulties, and regulatory barriers. They also require further research and development to prove their efficacy and feasibility.

The Importance of Early Intervention

Early intervention is the process of providing timely and appropriate services and support to people who are at risk of or experiencing the signs and symptoms of a neurodegenerative disease. Early intervention can have many benefits for the affected person and their caregivers, such as:

- Improving the accuracy and timeliness of diagnosis, prognosis, and monitoring of the disease
- Enhancing cognitive function and resilience and delaying or preventing cognitive decline or dementia
- Reducing the symptoms, complications, and progression of the disease
- Increasing access to and adherence to effective and safe treatments and therapies

- Preserving the quality of life and well-being of the person and their caregivers
- Reducing the social and economic costs and burden of the disease

It is crucial to take action early if you or anyone you know is worried about the progression or effects of a neurodegenerative disorder. By intervening early, it may be possible to alter the course and outcome of the disease and increase the likelihood of a more positive future.

Chapter 7

Lifestyle Interventions and Supportive Care

Exercise and Physical Therapy

Exercise and physical therapy are two types of lifestyle interventions that can help people with neurodegenerative diseases improve their brain function and quality of life. Exercise and physical therapy can have various benefits, such as:

- Improving blood flow, oxygen delivery, glucose metabolism, and neuroplasticity in the brain, which can enhance cognitive function and resilience and delay or prevent cognitive decline or dementia.

- Reducing the symptoms, complications, and progression of the disease, such as tremors, rigidity, slowness of movement, balance problems, muscle weakness, or spasticity.

- Increasing access and adherence to effective and safe treatments and therapies, such as medications, immunotherapy, or gene therapy, by improving the physical and mental health of the patient.

- Preserving the quality of life and well-being of the patient and their caregivers by boosting mood, self-esteem, and mental health and reducing stress, depression, and anxiety.

Exercise and physical therapy can take various forms, such as aerobic exercise, resistance training, balance training, stretching, or functional training. The type, intensity, frequency, and duration of exercise and physical therapy can vary depending on the type and stage of the disease, the availability and accessibility of the intervention, and the preference and compliance of the patient.

Therefore, it is important to consult with a medical professional before starting, changing, or stopping any exercise or physical therapy program for neurodegenerative diseases. Exercise and physical therapy are promising and effective lifestyle interventions that can help people with neurodegenerative diseases improve their brain function and quality of life.

Nutrition and Diet

Nutrition and diet are two types of lifestyle interventions that can help people with neurodegenerative diseases improve their brain function and quality of life. Nutrition and diet can have various benefits, such as:

- Providing the brain with essential nutrients, antioxidants, and anti-inflammatory compounds, which can enhance cognitive function and resilience and delay or prevent cognitive decline or dementia.
- Reducing the risk factors and complications of the disease, such as cardiovascular and

cerebrovascular diseases, diabetes, obesity, or metabolic syndrome, which can damage the brain and contribute to neurodegeneration.

- Increasing access and adherence to effective and safe treatments and therapies, such as medications, immunotherapy, or gene therapy, by improving the physical and mental health of the patient.
- Preserving the quality of life and well-being of the patient and their caregivers by boosting mood, self-esteem, and mental health and reducing stress, depression, and anxiety.

Nutrition and diet can take various forms, such as specific foods, natural supplements, or diet plans. Some of the foods and supplements that have been suggested for their neuroprotective properties are walnuts, omega-3 fatty acids, vitamin D, polyphenols, and probiotics.

Some of the diet plans that have been associated with a lower risk of neurodegenerative diseases are the Mediterranean diet, the ketogenic diet, and the MIND diet. The type, amount, and combination of nutrition and diet can vary depending on the type and stage of the disease, the availability and accessibility of the intervention, and the preference and compliance of the patient.

Supportive Care and Services

Supportive care and services are types of interventions that aim to provide emotional, social, and practical support to people with neurodegenerative diseases and their caregivers. Supportive care and services can have various benefits, such as:

- Improving the communication and relationship between the patient, the caregiver, and the healthcare team.
- Enhancing the coping skills and resilience of the patient and the caregiver and reducing stress, depression, and anxiety.
- Addressing the unmet needs and preferences of the patient and the caregiver, such as information, education, or resources.

- Providing comfort, dignity, and quality of life to the patient and the caregiver, especially in the end-of-life stage.

Supportive care and services can take various forms, such as counseling, education, coaching, support groups, or complementary therapies. The type, intensity, frequency, and duration of supportive care and services can vary depending on the type and stage of the disease, the availability and accessibility of the intervention, and the preference and compliance of the patient and the caregiver.

Chapter 8

Supporting Those with Neurodegenerative Diseases

Caregiving Strategies

Caring for someone with a neurodegenerative disease poses unique physical, emotional, and logistical challenges. Effective caregiving requires understanding the progressive nature of these illnesses, practicing patience, and prioritizing self-care. Tailoring strategies to the stage of the disease can help maximize patient function and maintain caregiver resilience.

Early on, focusing on safety-proofing the home, establishing routines, and encouraging independence fosters confidence. Simple memory aids like calendars, to-do lists, and medication dispensers support mild cognitive impairment. Normalizing the use of canes and walkers prevents falls as mobility declines.

In mid-stage disease, adapting activities to evolving capabilities is key. Simplifying tasks into step-by-step instructions accommodates processing impediments. Providing verbal cues or demonstrations taps into retained procedural memory. Engaging in creative arts, exercise, or music brings joy and preserves identity.

Later on, caregivers help compensate for significant cognitive and functional disabilities. Assisting with activities of daily living like bathing, dressing, and feeding maintains dignity. Simplifying communication using short phrases or non-verbal interactions bridges comprehension gaps.

Throughout the disease course, caregivers must also attend to their own mental and physical health through regular breaks, counseling, and respite support. Joining caregiver groups reduces isolation and provides solidarity. To share caregiving duties, it is essential to utilize the support of family and community.

Caregiving for neurodegenerative diseases demands tremendous patience, adaptability, and compassion. But small daily victories, like inspiring a smile or laugh, provide rewards along the challenging journey. Maintaining hopes and dreams for the future, however modest, lends meaning when disease robs much away.

Above all, well-informed caregivers can optimize quality of life through a responsive, patient-centered approach. Understanding the emotional impact of the disease allows caregivers to become the voice when patients can no longer advocate for themselves. With dedication and self-care, family caregivers impart invaluable comfort and dignity.

Maintaining Quality of Life

Neurodegenerative diseases erode function, independence, and identity. Yet, despite profound losses, much can be done to enrich the quality of life. Maintaining meaningful activities, social connections, and dignity can sustain purpose and hope even amid advanced disease.

Participating in hobbies and creative pursuits adapted to match current capabilities preserves a sense of joy and accomplishment. Caregivers can simplify steps for activities like cooking, puzzles, or art to accommodate disabilities while retaining the enriching aspects.

Music enhances mood and quality of life for both patients and caregivers. Singing your favorite old songs or learning new instruments stimulates cognition and reduces anxiety and agitation. Dancing, though adapted for wheelchairs or walkers, promotes movement.

Humor and laughter also carry healing power. Watching comedies together lifts spirits for all and strengthens social bonds. When possible, allowing patients to maintain their innate sense of humor gives comfort.

Support groups build solidarity and community for both people with neurodegenerative diseases and their caregivers. Sharing stories and creative techniques helps overcome isolation and loneliness.

Maintaining spiritual practices, adapted as needed, provides meaning and comfort through reflection and rituals. Nature experiences, like visiting parks or gardens, soothe the spirit. Touch therapies like massage ease restlessness while conveying warmth and caring.

Even simple pleasures, like enjoying favorite foods and music, watching beloved movies or TV shows, looking at family photo albums, or sitting outdoors, tap into positive memories and sensations. Finding daily opportunities for uplifting sensory experiences enriches time despite losses.

With family support and insights into patients' unique needs and wishes, people can craft fulfilling days even with neurodegenerative diseases. While these illnesses progress and eventually prove fatal, human bonds and simple joys sustain purpose each day. Focusing on enriching the present moment, however modestly, helps make the most of the remaining time and abilities.

Legal and Financial Planning

Receiving a neurodegenerative disease diagnosis prompts planning for future legal and financial needs before cognition declines. Addressing key issues early optimizes quality of life and provides peace of mind.

Establishing legal documents like advance directives for healthcare and durable powers of attorney is crucial. These allow designated, trusted people to make medical and financial decisions when patients cannot. Documents should be prepared before a significant impairment arises.

Designating powers of attorney helps ensure financial management aligns with values if judgment falters. Estate planning tools like wills and trusts distribute assets upon death as intended.

Memory impairment can endanger bill payment and credit, making automatic bill payment or consolidated account management prudent. Simplifying finances ahead of time preserves independence.

Determining care preferences via documents like Five Wishes guides comfort, food, visitors, and personal care. Outlining wishes for quality of life if hospitalization occurs is wise.

Forecasting care costs helps calculate the required savings and insurance coverage. Long-term care insurance merits consideration for covering home care, assisted living, or nursing facilities. Consulting elder law attorneys navigates complex financial matters.

Exploring community resources locates appropriate housing, respite, transportation, and support services. Familiarizing yourself with options before intensive needs arise enables smooth transitions later.

Initiating end-of-life conversations within families ensures that care is aligned with patients' values when they lack decision-making capacity.

While neurodegenerative disease brings profound uncertainty, future-oriented planning restores a sense of control. By thoughtfully arranging legal and financial matters during capacity, patients secure their wishes for health, family, and assets. This lifts burdens from loved ones during difficult times ahead. With foresight and courageous conversations, families gain comfort and closure.

Communication Tips

Communicating effectively with someone experiencing progressive neurocognitive impairment requires patience, creativity, and compassion. Adapting approaches to the person's unique needs and deficits sustains engagement and understanding.

Speak slowly in short, simple sentences to aid comprehension. Allow ample time for responses. Eliminate distractions and make full eye contact to help focus attention.

Use orienting cues like names, dates, and places to provide context. Write down keywords to reinforce the main ideas. Keep instructions concrete and step-by-step.

When word-finding falters, provide gentle suggestions or fill in the gaps. Avoid quizzing. Instead, make the conversation light and relaxed. Bring in notes or photos to illustrate stories.

Allow the person to communicate through whatever means they can, whether speaking, writing, pointing, or gesturing. Verify understanding by summarizing or repeating key points.

To ease anxiety, offer reassurance through calm tones and comforting body language. Acknowledge the feelings behind words or behaviors. Distraction and redirection work better than arguing.

Caregivers can foster meaningful engagement by sharing news, music, poetry, or religious passages. Looking at photo albums together allows individuals to draw on an intact long-term memory.

Laughing together strengthens bonds when used sensitively. Humor relieves stress and discomfort. Focus on the positives and the joy of being present together.

Above all, maintain dignity and personhood. Avoid talking down, correcting, or scolding. Uphold adult roles and use the person's preferred name. Honor the individual's reality to build trust.

Despite profound memory loss, engagement and expression remain possible with creative, compassionate communication. Relating to the preserved essence of the person beneath the disease symptoms conveys respect and care through the difficult journey.

Conclusion

As we have seen throughout this introductory guide, neurodegenerative diseases pose a formidable threat to the health of our brains and nervous systems. The progressive and debilitating nature of conditions like Alzheimer's and Parkinson's disease underscores the need for increased research efforts and medical advancements.

While there are no cures yet, scientists are piecing together the complex neurological puzzles posed by these disorders. Though neurodegeneration cannot yet be reversed or definitively prevented, the treatments and lifestyle changes outlined in this book can significantly improve quality of life and slow symptom progression.

Early intervention is key, as lasting damage can occur before obvious signs appear. However, better long-term prognoses are possible by staying attuned to subtle cognitive or motor changes, seeking prompt medical advice, and considering emerging therapies like immunotherapy.

While caring for someone with neurocognitive decline is undoubtedly challenging, we explored tips for preserving dignity and engagement at each stage through thoughtful caregiving approaches. Many legal, financial, and healthcare resources are also available to provide further support. With a combination of medical treatment, lifestyle changes, caregiver support, and advances in research, the future looks brighter for those facing neurodegenerative disease.

By learning about where we stand today in understanding, diagnosing, and treating these disorders, we empower ourselves to face the changes ahead with knowledge, resources, and hope. Though mystery still surrounds many aspects of diseases like Alzheimer's and Parkinson's, progress is steady.

The passionate work of doctors, scientists, and advocates is moving us ever closer to uncovering effective means of detecting, managing, and preventing neurodegeneration.

References

---

1. Alzheimer's Association. (2019). 2019 Alzheimer's disease facts and figures. Alzheimer's & Dementia, 15(3), 321-387. https://doi.org/10.1016/j.jalz.2019.01.010

2. Cohen, A. (2018). Caregiving for a loved one with dementia: If only I knew then what I know now. Jessica Kingsley Publishers.

3. Jack, C.R., Bennett, D.A., Blennow, K., Carrillo, M.C., Feldman, H.H., Frisoni, G.B., Hampel, H., Jagust, W.J., Johnson, K.A., Knopman, D.S., Petersen, R.C., Scheltens, P., Sperling, R.A., & Dubois, B. (2016). A/T/N: An unbiased descriptive classification scheme for Alzheimer's disease biomarkers. Neurology, 87(5), 539-547. https://doi.org/10.1212/WNL.00000000000 02923.

Resources

Here are resources that you can use to learn more about neurodegenerative diseases and their treatment:

- [Neurodegenerative Diseases: What They Are & Types - Cleveland Clinic](https://my.clevelandclinic.org/health/diseases/17827-neurodegenerative-diseases)
- [Neurodegenerative Diseases - National Institute of Environmental Health Sciences](https://www.niehs.nih.gov/health/topics/conditions/neurodegenerative/index.cfm)
- [The Path Forward: Advancing Treatments and Cures for Neurodegenerative Diseases](https://www.fastercures.org/assets

/Uploads/Neurodegenerative-Diseases-Repor t.pdf)

- [Solving neurodegeneration: common mechanisms and strategies for new therapies](https://www.nature.com/articles/ s41586-021-03594-0)
- [Neurodegenerative Disease: Improving Outcomes Through Nutrition](https://www.todaysdietitian.com/ newarchives/0320p24.shtml)
- [Preventive and Therapeutic Potential of Physical Exercise in Neurodegenerative Diseases](https://www.frontiersin.org/article s/10.3389/fnins.2017.00688/full)
- [Frontiers | Supportive care of neurodegenerative patients](https://www.frontiersin.org/resear ch-topics/14661/supportive-care-of-neurodeg enerative-patients)
- [Alzheimer's Association | Alzheimer's Disease & Dementia Help](https://www.alz.org/)

- [Parkinson's Foundation: Better Lives. Together.](https://www.parkinson.org/)
- [ALS Association](http://www.alsa.org/)
- [Huntington's Disease Society of America](https://hdsa.org/)
- [National Multiple Sclerosis Society: Home](https://www.nationalmssociety.org/)